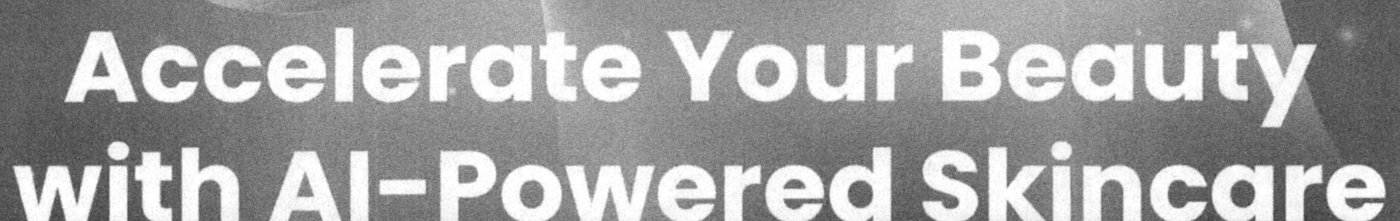

Accelerate Your Beauty with AI-Powered Skincare

This book unveils the pioneering innovations shaping the future of skincare, positioning readers at the forefront of this exciting paradigm shift.

Anna Chacon Dermatologist, MD USA

Josef Namin

Healthcare IT Integration Architect

Ac

celerate your Beauty with AI-powered Skincare

Josef Namin

Table of contents

Introduction

What is Artificial Intelligence (AI):

Artificial Intelligence, commonly known as AI, is the simulation of human intelligence processes by machines, especially computer systems. These processes include learning (acquiring information and rules for using the information), reasoning (using rules to reach approximate or definitive conclusions), and self-correction. Over the years, AI has spread through various sectors, transforming how we operate and interact with technology.

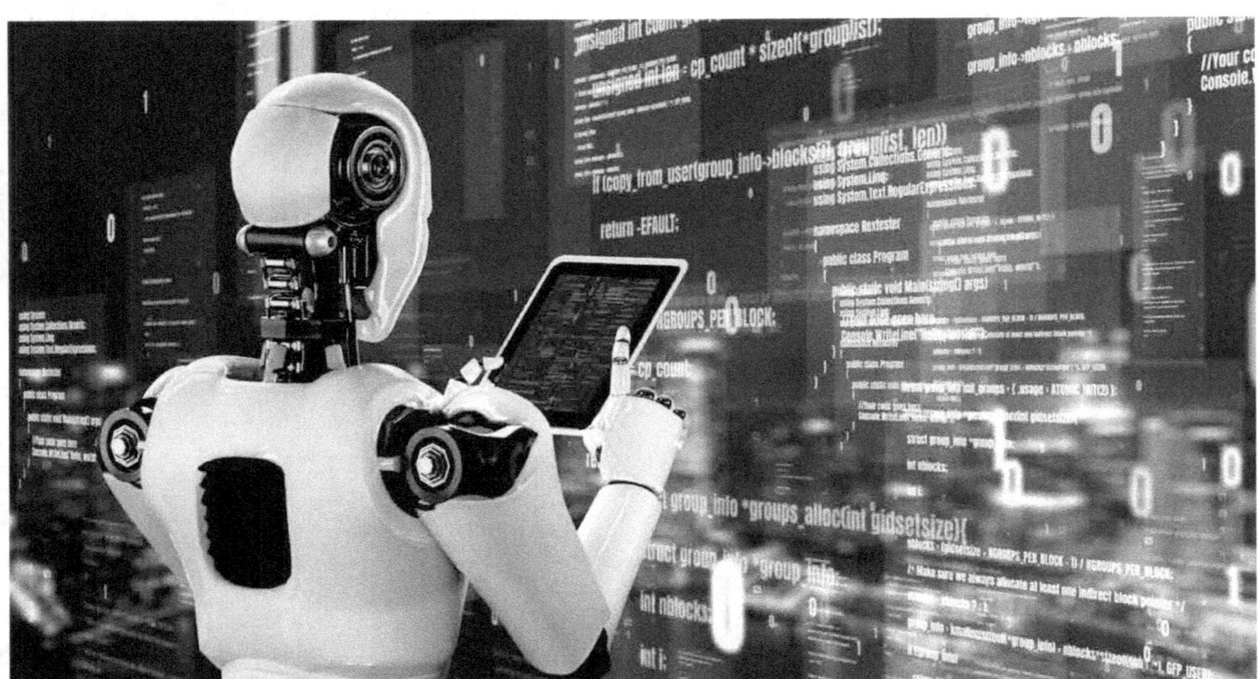

What is AI-powered skincare?

AI-powered skincare uses artificial intelligence to develop products and technologies that are more effective, personalized, and efficient. It refers to the integration of Artificial Intelligence into skincare products, routines, and diagnostics. AI can offer personalized skincare recommendations, predict skin health trends, and even create tailor-made products by analyzing vast datasets about skin types, conditions, and effective treatments. This fusion of technology and personal care promises a revolution in how we approach our skincare.

Evolution of Beauty Tech

Beauty has been at the forefront of technological innovation for many years. From the invention of the first lipstick in 3500 BC to the development of laser hair removal in the 1980s, beauty brands have consistently embraced new technologies to improve their products and treatments.

AI has emerged as one of the most transformative technologies in the beauty industry in recent years. The introduction of technology into the beauty space began with basic tools and has now expanded to sophisticated devices and software. With the dawn of AI, the beauty technology landscape has experienced exponential growth in innovation, offering remarkable solutions and products tailored to individual needs.

AI is also being used to develop and formulate new skincare products and ingredients. For example, AI-powered systems are being used to design new peptides and other active ingredients that are more effective at targeting specific skin conditions.

AI is also being used to create new beauty experiences. For example, AR (Augmented reality) and VR (Virtual Reality) apps now allow consumers to virtually try makeup and skincare products before purchasing them.

The evolution of beauty technology is being driven by a number of factors, including:
- **Consumer demand:** Consumers are increasingly demanding personalized and effective skincare products. AI is able to meet this demand by providing consumers with personalized recommendations and by tracking their progress over time.
- **Technological advancements:** AI technology is rapidly advancing, making it possible to develop AI-powered skincare systems that are more accurate and effective than ever before.
- **Investment from beauty brands:** Beauty brands are investing heavily in AI research and development. This investment is helping to accelerate the development of new AI-powered skincare products and technologies.

The evolution of beauty technology is having a significant impact on the way we care for our skin. AI-powered skincare systems are making it possible for us to achieve our skincare goals more effectively and efficiently than ever before.

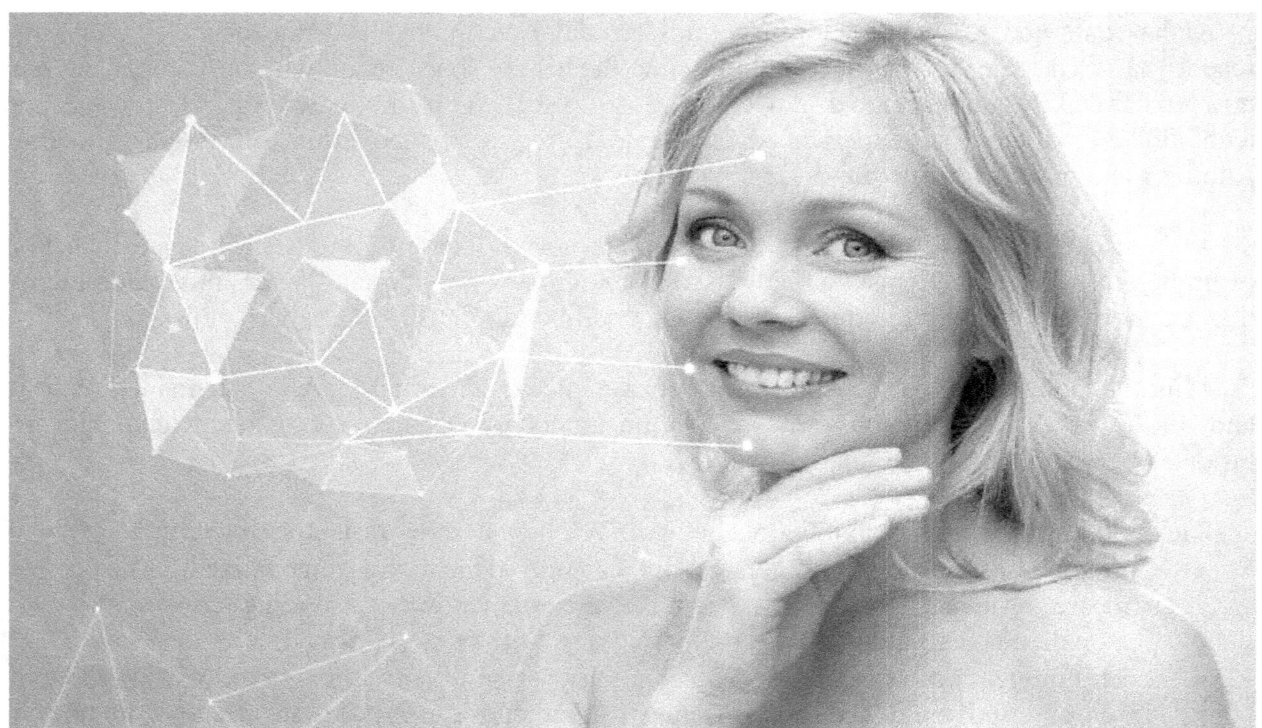

Chapter 1

The Rise of AI in Personal Care & Beauty

How does AI function in skincare?

AI's functionality in skincare revolves around its ability to process vast amounts of data at lightning speed. It can assess millions of skin profiles, noting patterns and discrepancies. This enables AI to offer solutions catered to individual skin profiles.

Detecting different skin types: Utilizing advanced algorithms, AI can scan and analyze facial images to distinguish between skin types. Whether someone has oily, dry, combination, or normal skin, AI tools can often identify these characteristics more accurately than the human eye.

Identifying common skin concerns: From acne and rosacea to fine lines and hyperpigmentation, AI can identify common skin problems by analyzing skin patterns, colors, and textures, thus aiding in the recommendation of appropriate treatments, making it easier for healthcare professionals and dermatologists as well to tailor the treatment according to the requirements of the patient

Benefits of using AI-powered skincare

AI-powered skincare systems offer a number of benefits, including:

- **Personalization:** AI can help you create a skincare regimen tailored specifically to your unique skin type and concerns.
- **Accuracy:** AI systems can analyze your skin more accurately than the human eye because even dermatologists need tools to examine the skin with a magnifying device and good lighting to illuminate the area to be examined. Therefore, AI can identify even the most subtle changes that an unaided human eye can miss
- **Convenience:** AI-powered skincare systems are easy to use and can provide personalized recommendations in seconds.
- **Affordability:** AI-powered skincare systems are becoming increasingly affordable because they save you from a private consultation, making them accessible to a broader range of consumers.

The infusion of digital tools in beauty:

The infusion of digital tools in beauty is also accelerating the adoption of AI-powered skincare. From AR-powered virtual makeup trials to mobile apps that track skin health over time, the combination of digital tools with beauty has made the skincare and makeup industry more interactive, customizable, and user-centric than ever before.

Case Study: AI in Action - Neutrogena's Personalized Skincare Revolution

In an industry where one-size-fits-all solutions often fall short, Neutrogena, a well-known skincare brand, embarked on a groundbreaking journey to harness the power of Artificial Intelligence (AI) to revolutionize personalized skincare. This case study provides an in-depth look into how Neutrogena has successfully employed AI to lead a skincare revolution.

- **AI-Powered Skin Analysis for Unprecedented Precision:**

Neutrogena recognized the need for a more precise approach to skincare that truly understood each individual's unique skin needs. To achieve this, they introduced an AI-driven skin analysis tool accessible via the Neutrogena website and mobile app. Users simply uploaded a photo of their face, and the AI algorithms, driven by deep learning and computer vision, meticulously examined the image. This comprehensive analysis enabled the system to determine skin type, identify specific concerns such as fine lines, wrinkles, or uneven tone, and evaluate hydration levels.

- **Personalized Skincare Recommendations Tailored to Perfection:**

Armed with this detailed analysis, Neutrogena's AI system generated highly personalized skincare recommendations. These recommendations are factored into the user's individual skin profile, lifestyle, and product preferences. The AI not only suggested the most suitable products from Neutrogena's extensive range but also provided guidance on their optimal usage. Furthermore, the system considered environmental factors like the user's location and current weather conditions, ensuring that the skincare routine remained effective and adaptable.

- **Real-Time Skin Monitoring for Continual Improvement:**

Neutrogena didn't stop at initial recommendations. They introduced a real-time skin monitoring feature, allowing users to track the progress of their skincare journey over time. By regularly submitting updated photos and data, users could witness firsthand the positive transformations in their skin. The AI system adapted its recommendations in response to evolving skin conditions, ensuring that users continually received the most effective and relevant guidance.

- **Elevated Customer Engagement and Satisfied Users:**

The results of Neutrogena's AI-driven approach were truly remarkable. Users reported significantly higher satisfaction levels with their skincare routines, coupled with a noticeable reduction in common skin issues. Customers' engagement with the brand soared as they experienced the benefits of personalized care. Neutrogena successfully built a community of loyal customers who valued the brand's commitment to their unique beauty needs.

For more information about the Neutrogena AI system, please visit the following link: https://skin360.neutrogena.com

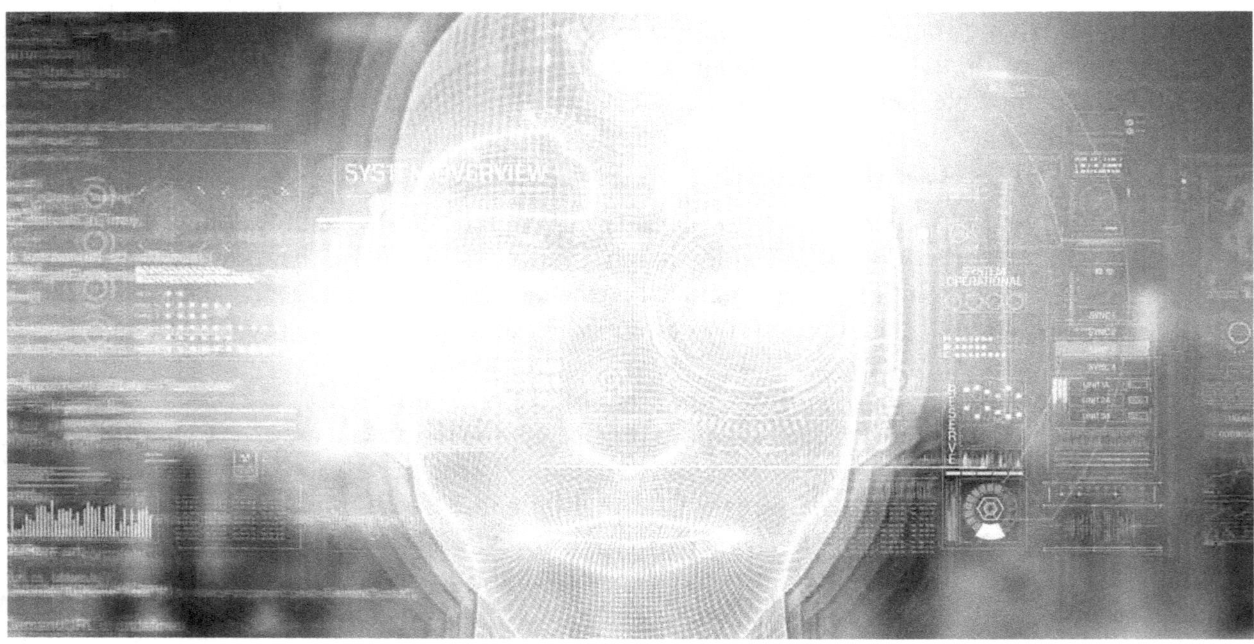

Chapter 2

AI-Powered Skincare Products and Technologies

Current Applications of AI in the Beauty Industry

AI's footprint in the beauty industry is vast and growing. It has transformed various aspects of beauty, making it more personalized and tech-centric. There are a number of different types of

AI-powered skincare products and technologies available today. Some of the most common include:

- **AI in product formulation:** AI is now employed in laboratories, analyzing countless ingredients and their interactions, resulting in optimized product formulations that cater to a wide range of skin needs.
- **Virtual assistants in beauty shopping:** Chatbots and virtual assistants, powered by AI, guide users through online shopping experiences, answering queries and offering product recommendations based on individual preferences.
- **Predictive analytics for future beauty trends:** By analyzing current trends, user feedback, and market dynamics, AI tools can predict upcoming beauty trends, allowing brands to stay ahead of the curve.

Different types of AI-powered skincare products and technologies:

- From smart mirrors that analyze skin health in real-time to devices that customize serums and creams based on skin's daily needs, AI-powered products and technology tools are varied. These innovations offer consumers a futuristic approach to skincare, where devices not only advise but also adapt to changing skin needs.

How to choose and use the right AI-powered skincare products

As with any product, selecting AI-powered skincare devices and technologies that align with one's unique skin needs is essential. By understanding the technology behind a product, checking user reviews, and consulting dermatologists or skincare professionals, users can ensure that they're making informed choices.

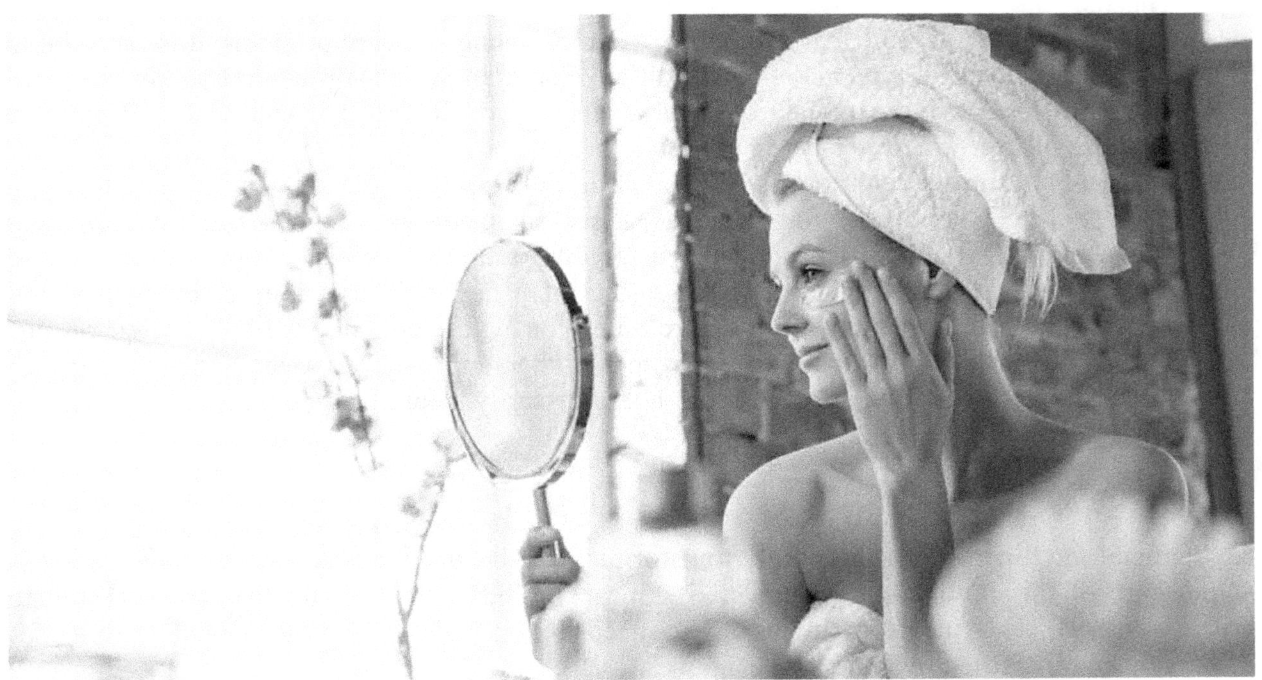

Chapter 3

Personalizing Your Skincare with AI

How to assess your skin type and concerns

AI can help you personalize your skincare routine in several ways. For example, you can use an AI-powered skin analysis tool to identify your skin type and concerns. You can then use this information to choose the right skincare products and develop a skin care regimen tailored to your specific needs.

Identifying skin type and understanding particular concerns are the foundational steps in any effective skincare regimen. While traditional methods involve manual assessments and quizzes, AI-powered tools now offer digital assessments, analyzing facial photographs or real-time scans to provide detailed skin analyses.

Developing a personalized AI-powered skincare routine

Here are some tips for developing a personalized AI-powered skincare routine:

1. **Start with a clean foundation:** Before developing a personalized skincare regimen, start with a clean foundation, which means cleansing your face with a gentle cleanser.
2. **Use an AI-powered skin analysis tool:** An AI-powered skin analysis tool can help you identify your skin type and concerns. Once you know your skin type and concerns, you can choose the right skincare products and develop a routine tailored to your specific skin needs.
3. **Choose the right skincare products:** When choosing skincare products, it is essential to consider your skin type and skin condition. For example, if you have dry skin, you will want to choose more moisturizing products. If you have oily skin, you will want to choose oil-free and water-based products.
4. **Develop a simple regimen:** It is essential to develop a simple skincare routine that you can stick to. Start with a few basic steps, such as cleansing, moisturizing, and applying sunscreen. You can add additional steps to your routine as needed.
5. **Be patient:** It takes time to see the results of a new skincare routine. Be patient and consistent with your daily skincare routine; you will eventually see the desired results. Remember that every person differs from the other, so if your relative or friend has gotten the same results in one month, it does not necessarily mean that you will be achieving the same results at the same time.

Case Studies: Brands that excel in personalized AI interactions.

Artificial intelligence (AI) is rapidly transforming the beauty industry, and personalization is at the core of this revolution. AI-powered skincare brands use data and machine learning to create personalized skincare regimens for each customer. This is leading to better results for customers and increased revenue for businesses.

Here are a few case studies of brands that excel in personalized AI interactions:

HiMirror

HiMirror is a smart beauty mirror that uses AI to analyze the skin and provide personalized skincare recommendations. The HiMirror comes with a variety of other features, such as a virtual makeup try-on tool and a skin-tracking system.

L'Oréal Paris

L'Oréal Paris offers a variety of AI-powered skincare products and services. For example, the L'Oréal Paris Magic Modista app uses AI to analyze clients' faces and recommend makeup looks tailored to their specific facial features. L'Oréal Paris also offers a personalized skincare service called My Skin Advisor, which uses AI to analyze the customer's skin and recommend skincare products.

Neutrogena

Neutrogena offers a variety of AI-powered skincare services, such as the Neutrogena Skin360 app and the Neutrogena Skin360 Analyzer. The Skin360 app allows clients to take selfies and track their skin's progress over time. The Skin360 Analyzer is a handheld device that takes images of the skin and uses AI to analyze them for signs of aging, sun damage, and other skin conditions.

Personalized AI interactions

These are just a few examples of brands that are using AI to deliver personalized experiences to their clients. As AI technology continues to evolve, we expect to see even more innovative and effective ways to use AI for personalized skincare treatment and care.

Here are some of the ways that these brands are using AI to deliver personalized interactions:

- **Using AI to analyze customer data:** These brands use AI to analyze customer data, such as purchase history, skin type, and skin concerns, to develop personalized recommendations.
- **Using AI to create interactive experiences:** These brands use AI to create interactive experiences, such as virtual makeup try-ons and skin tracking systems, that allow customers to explore different skincare options and see the results in real time.
- **Using AI to provide personalized support:** These brands use AI to provide personalized support to their customers, such as answering questions and offering advice.

Tips for maximizing the benefits of your AI-powered skincare regimen:

- Embracing AI in skincare is not just about using the technology but optimizing its benefits. Regularly updating AI tools based on feedback, consistently following the recommended routine, and staying informed about the latest AI skincare advancements can help users derive the maximum value from their AI-powered skincare journey.

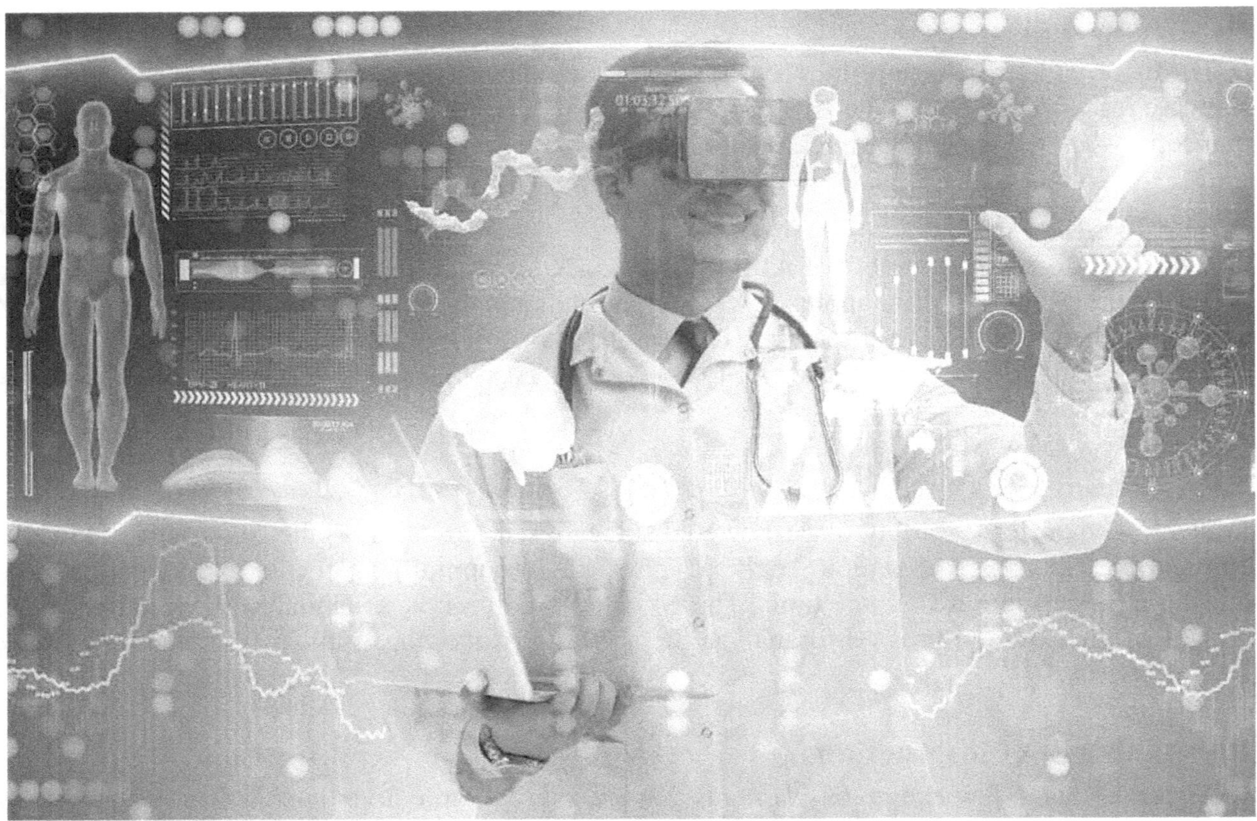

Chapter 4

The Role of AR and VR in Beauty

How AR Transforms Beauty Product Trials

Augmented Reality (AR) has redefined product trials in the beauty industry. Instead of physically applying a product, users can now virtually "try on" makeup or hairstyles using AR filters, providing a no-mess, commitment-free experience that allows them to experiment with countless looks in seconds. This can help them find the right products for their skin type and tone and avoid wasting money on products they don't like or do not suit them.

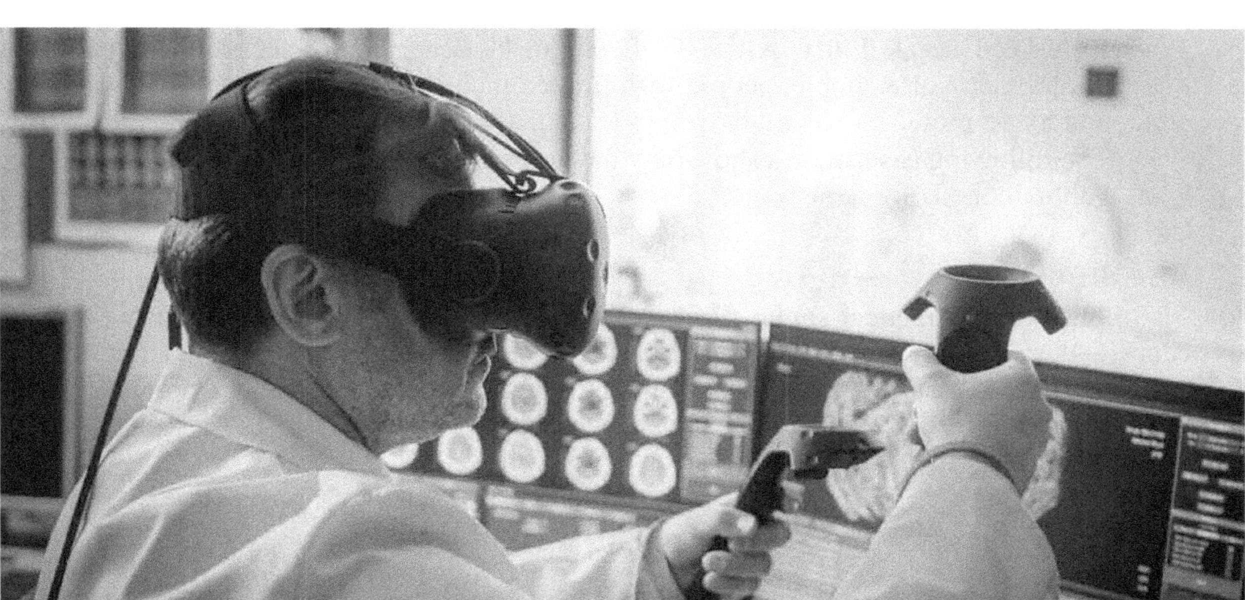

Virtual Reality (VR) in Beauty Experiences

In the ever-evolving landscape of the beauty industry, Virtual Reality (VR) has emerged as a game-changer, offering consumers immersive beauty experiences like never before. VR goes beyond mere product try-ons; it transports users into virtual spa and salon environments, where they can indulge in relaxation and self-care from the comfort of their homes. VR is reshaping how consumers engage with beauty products and services, whether it's virtually trying out different hairstyles, exploring skincare treatments, or even immersing oneself in a tranquil spa day. By simulating real-world beauty experiences, VR not only provides consumers with a sense of control and exploration but also offers beauty brands a unique avenue for engaging and connecting with their customers on a deeper, more personal level.

Augmented Reality (AR) vs. Virtual Reality (VR) in Beauty

While both AR and Virtual Reality (VR) offer immersive technology experiences, they serve different purposes in beauty. AR overlays digital information in the real world, facilitating virtual makeup trials or skincare simulations. In contrast, VR offers a fully immersive digital environment, which can be utilized for virtual spa treatments or exploring virtual beauty stores.

Benefits of AR try-ons: Sustainability, inclusivity, and enhanced accessibility:
- AR not only offers convenience but also addresses more significant industry concerns. Virtual try-ons reduce product waste, as clients no longer need physical samples for every trial.
- **Sustainability:** AR and VR can help to reduce waste in the beauty industry by allowing consumers to try on products before they buy them.
- **Inclusivity:** AR and VR can help make beauty more inclusive by allowing consumers to try on products that are not available in their local stores or designed for their skin type or tone.

- **Enhanced accessibility:** AR and VR can make beauty more accessible to people with disabilities. For example, people with limited mobility can use VR to visit beauty stores and try on products without having to leave their homes.
- The following case studies show how the usage of AR and VR is constantly increasing in public in the US:

Case Studies: Successful Implementations of AR in Beauty

To illustrate the practical applications and success stories of Augmented Reality (AR) in the beauty industry, this section highlights several noteworthy case studies. These examples showcase how AR has revolutionized how consumers interact with beauty products and how brands have leveraged this technology to enhance user experiences.

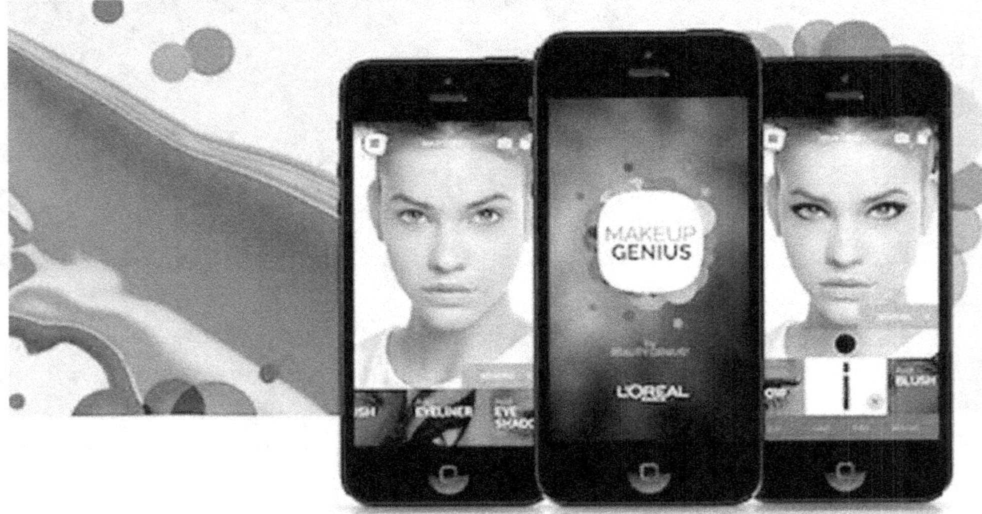

L'Oreal's AR Beauty App:

L'Oreal, a global beauty giant, introduced an AR beauty app that allows users to virtually try on various makeup products in real time using their smartphones or tablets. By simply scanning their face through the app, consumers can experiment with different shades of lipstick, eyeshadow, and foundation. The app's sophisticated AR technology accurately maps facial features, ensuring the virtual makeup looks realistic and aligns with individual skin tones. L'Oreal's AR beauty app not only offers a risk-free way for customers to explore their products but also provides valuable data on consumer preferences, aiding the company in tailoring their product offerings.

For more information, please visit the following link:
https://www.loreal.com/en/articles/science-and-technology/makeup-virtual-try-on-maybelline/

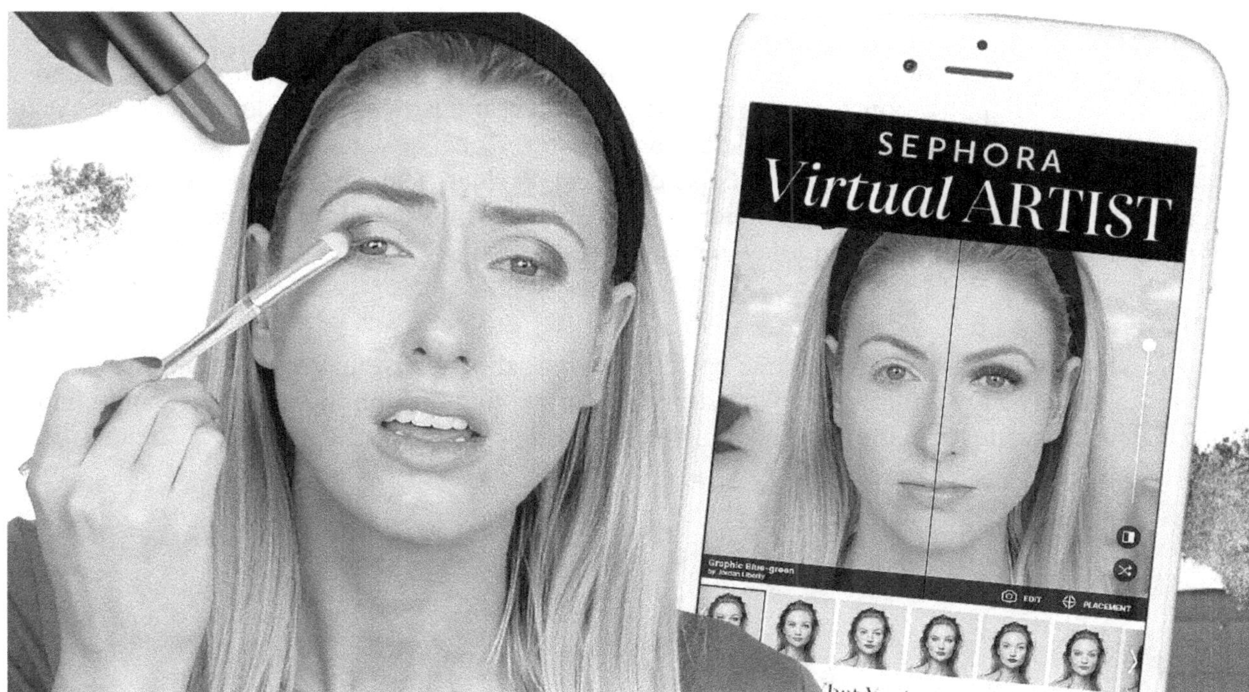

Sephora's Virtual Artist:

Sephora, a leading beauty retailer, introduced the "Virtual Artist" feature within its app, which utilizes AR to allow customers to try on a vast array of makeup products virtually. Users can see how various shades and products would look on their own faces, providing an interactive and informative shopping experience. Sephora's Virtual Artist has not only boosted customer engagement but also significantly reduced product returns, as consumers can confidently select the right products for their needs. These case studies highlight how AR has become an indispensable tool for beauty brands in enhancing customer satisfaction and driving sales through immersive and personalized experiences.

For more information, please visit the following link:
https://www.sephora.my/pages/virtual-artist

Proven Skincare:

Proven Skincare is a consumer app that uses machine learning to create individual skincare regimens based on a customer's unique skin type. The company states that the recommended regimen is based on their Beauty Genome Project, a database of more than 8 million customer product reviews, 100,000 skincare products, and 20,000 ingredients, as well as information from scientific or peer-reviewed journal articles about skin and ingredients.

Coty:

Coty offers an augmented reality virtual mirror software called Magic Mirror. The Magic Mirror uses computed vision technology and was developed in collaboration with digital creative studio Holition and digital marketing company Perch Interactive. Coty claims the mirror allows customers to virtually wear products from its collection

ModiFace:

ModiFace offers augmented reality applications, including Skin AI, an anti-aging and skin care simulation application for the beauty and medical industries. The company claims that the video-based application is able to detect and quantify changes in the skin, as well as predict changes in the skin condition after the use of a skin product. The application was developed with the help of dermatologists to measure and assess skin conditions such as dark spots, discolorations, dryness, uneven tone, and fine wrinkles.

Perfect Corp. :

Perfect Corp. offers a smartphone application that allows customers to use augmented reality to test a variety of makeup looks. The company claims that the application uses a combination of face detection and tracking, augmented reality (AR), and live 3D Face AR to create different looks.

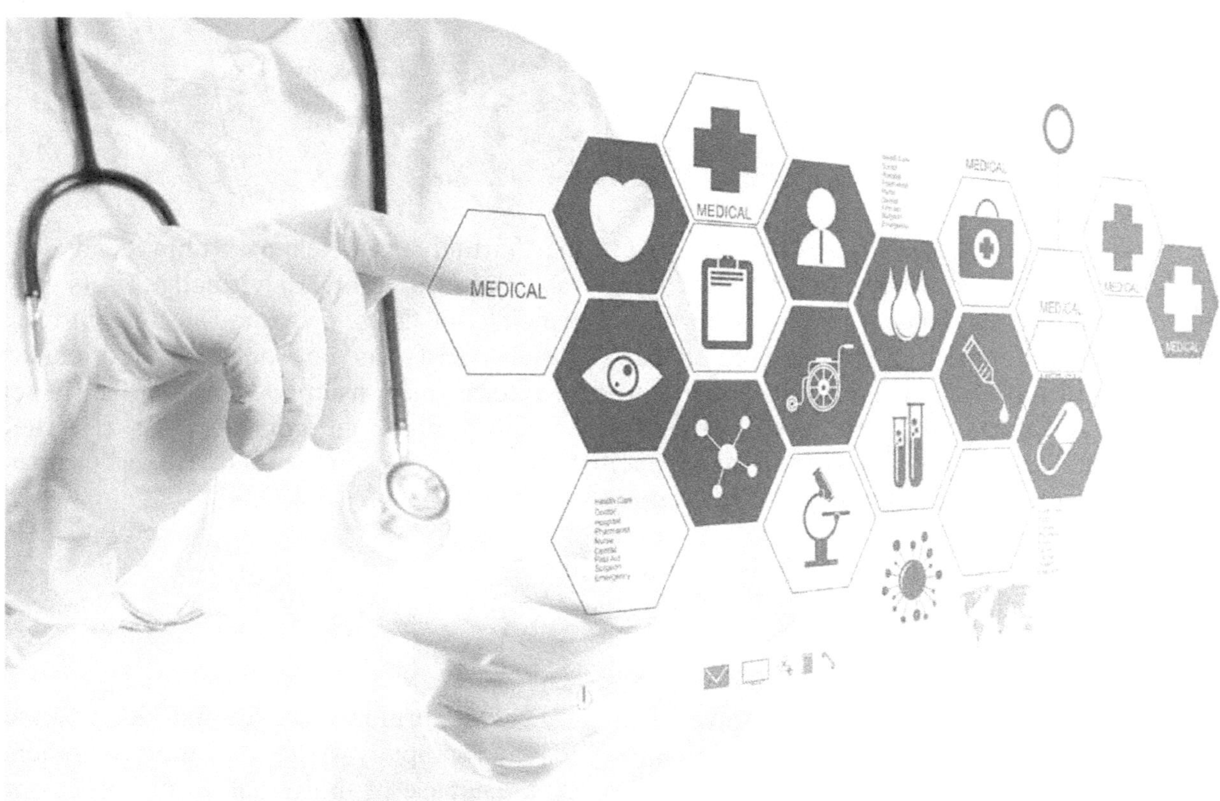

Chapter 5

The Future of AI in Personal Care

The shift towards personalized solutions using AI

The future of AI in personal care is very bright. AI is becoming increasingly sophisticated and affordable and being used to develop new and innovative skincare products and technologies.

- One of the most exciting trends in AI skincare is the development of personalized products and treatments. AI can be used to analyze the skin's unique needs and to develop products and treatments that are tailored to the individual skins needs. This could lead to a new era of personalized skincare that is more effective and efficient than ever before.
- AI is also being used to develop new ways to diagnose and treat skin conditions. For example, AI-powered systems are being developed to detect skin cancer early and to recommend personalized treatment options.
- Overall, the future of AI in personal care is very promising. AI has the potential to revolutionize the way we care for our skin.
- As AI tools become more sophisticated, they'll offer even more tailored skincare solutions, taking into account factors like genetics, diet, and lifestyle, ensuring that every individual's skincare routine is as unique as their fingerprint.
- Having said that, it is crucial to know that the development of these advancements associated with AI needs a dedicated team of dermatologists who have significant experience and expertise in their field and, at the same time, are keeping up with the recent advancements in technology as well.
- Here are some additional thoughts on the future of AI in dermatology:
- AI is likely to play an even more significant role in early skin cancer detection. AI systems are constantly being improved, and they are becoming better and better at identifying skin cancer in its early stages. This could lead to a significant reduction in the number of people who develop advanced skin cancer.
- AI is likely to be used to develop new and more effective treatments for skin conditions. AI can be used to screen millions of potential drug compounds to identify those most likely effective against specific skin conditions. This could lead to the development of new treatments that are more effective and have fewer side effects than current treatments.
- AI is likely to make dermatology care more accessible to everyone. AI chatbots and other AI-powered tools can provide patients with access to information and advice about skin conditions, even if they do not have access to a dermatologist. This could help to reduce health disparities and improve the quality of life for people with skin conditions.

Overall, the future of AI in dermatology is very bright. AI has the potential to revolutionize the way that skin conditions are diagnosed, treated, and managed.

AI's increasing relevance in daily skincare practices

Beyond specialized tools and devices, AI's integration into everyday skincare practices is imminent. From AI-powered smart mirrors that offer daily skin analyses to AI-driven mobile apps that adjust routines based on daily skin feedback, AI will soon become an inseparable part of our daily skincare rituals.

AI's potential to revolutionize skincare understanding and treatment:

AI not only promises better products but also a deeper understanding of the skin itself. By analyzing vast skin data, AI can unearth patterns and insights previously overlooked, potentially leading to breakthroughs in skincare treatments and even redefining our understanding of skin health.

The following report shows websites or stores that US beauty shoppers visit when searching for beauty products. Fewer than a third of US shoppers turn to department stores' websites (31%) or brick-and-mortar locations (24%) when conducting beauty research, according to a May survey conducted by PowerReviews. In contrast, 71% turn to a specialty retailer's website when researching new products.

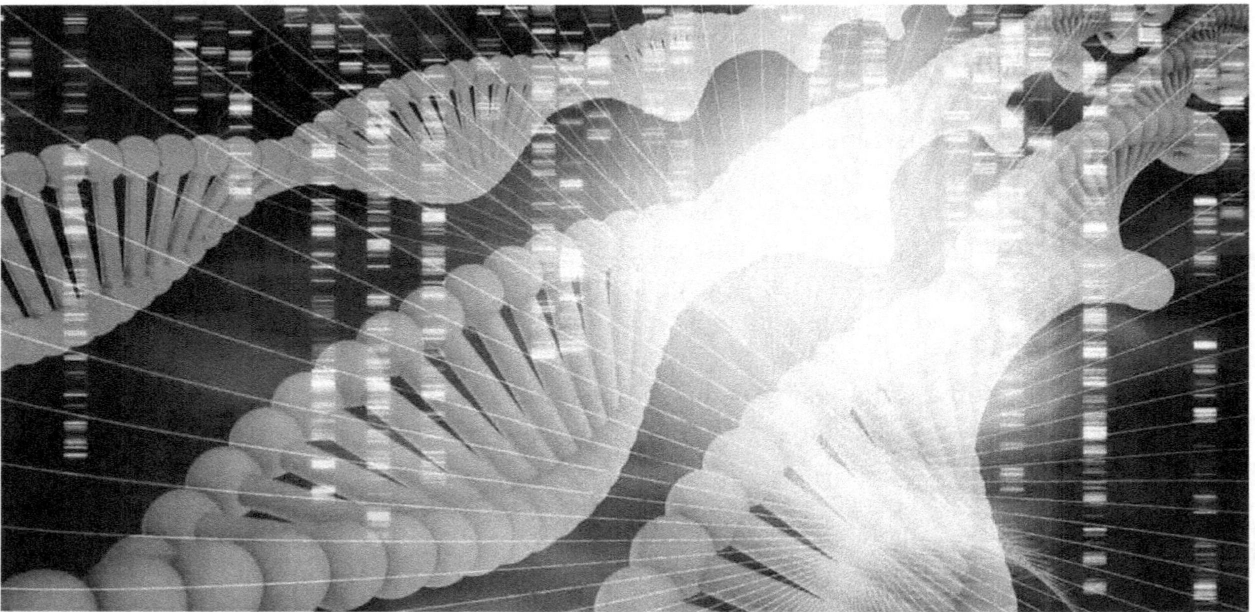

Chapter 6

Beyond Beauty: Biotech, AI, and Skincare Convergence

The intersections of various technologies in skincare

The future of skincare lies at the intersection of multiple technologies. Alongside AI, advancements in biotech, nanotechnology, and even quantum computing promise to redefine skincare's future landscape, offering solutions that seem straight out of science fiction today. For example, biotechnology is being used to develop new skincare ingredients that are more effective and less irritating. AI is being used to develop new ways to deliver these ingredients to the skin more effectively.

AI-powered skincare treatments:

AI-powered skincare treatments represent a fusion of cutting-edge technology and beauty science, offering promising solutions to address various skin concerns at their core. Let's embark on a journey that explores the potential of AI in revolutionizing skincare treatments, from laser therapies to gene editing.

- **AI-powered lasers and light therapies:** AI can be used to develop new lasers and light therapies that are more effective and less invasive. For example, AI can be used to develop lasers that can target specific skin concerns, such as scars, wrinkles, and acne.

- **AI-powered microneedling devices:** AI-powered microneedling devices can be used to deliver skincare ingredients into the skin more effectively. For example, AI can be used to control the depth and speed of the microneedling process to ensure that the skincare ingredients are delivered to the right layers of the skin, as the main purpose of microneedling is to rejuvenate the skin by stimulating collagen production.
- **AI-powered minimally invasive procedures:** AI can help dermatologists and aesthetic practitioners guide about the true and effective placement of dermal fillers and Botox. AI algorithms can analyze facial features and recommend the sites for the correct volume to be injected at specific areas of the face to prevent over-injection or undesired results.
- **AI-guided cosmetic surgery:** AI empowers plastic surgeons with real-time guidance during cosmetic procedures as well. By analyzing patient data, AI recommends surgical techniques tailored to the individual's face, body, and preferences, ensuring a natural and personalized outcome. This technology enhances precision and patient satisfaction in the field of cosmetic surgery.
- **AI-powered gene editing:** AI can be used to develop new gene editing techniques that can be used to treat skin conditions at the root cause as part of a holistic approach to health care and well being. For example, AI could be used to develop gene editing techniques that can be used to repair genes that are mutated in skin cancer.

Upcoming therapies: Genomics, nanotech, and more:

The next frontier in skincare treatments will leverage insights from genomics, the study of genes and their functions. Combined with nanotech's precision and AI's computational power, we might see treatments that are not only skin-deep but address the very genetic makeup of an individual.

The convergence of these technologies has the potential to revolutionize the skincare industry and to create new and innovative products that are more effective, efficient, and personalized than ever before.

Ethical and societal implications of bio-integrated beauty

As skincare technologies advance, they bring along ethical dilemmas. Bio-integrated beauty, where technology and biology merge, will necessitate a robust ethical framework. Issues like data privacy, genetic modifications, and societal perceptions of beauty will need thoughtful deliberation and regulation.

Case Study: L'Oréal Paris' Innovative Bio-Integrated Skincare

L'Oréal Paris is a leading skincare brand that is known for its innovative products and technologies. In recent years, L'Oréal Paris has begun to focus on developing bio-integrated skincare products. Bio-integrated skincare products are designed to work with the skin's natural biology to improve its appearance and health.

One of L'Oréal Paris' most innovative bio-integrated skincare products is the *Revitalift Bio-Peptide Day Cream*. This cream contains a blend of peptides and hyaluronic acid that work together to boost collagen production, reduce the appearance of wrinkles, and hydrate the skin.

Another innovative bio-integrated skincare product from L'Oréal Paris is the *Age Perfect Cell Renewal Night Serum*. This serum contains a blend of retinol, niacinamide, and hyaluronic acid that work together to exfoliate the skin, reduce the appearance of age spots, and even out the skin tone.

L'Oréal Paris is also developing new bio-integrated skincare technologies. For example, L'Oréal Paris is working on a new technology called "Skinimalism" that uses AI to create personalized skin care treatment regimens with only the essential products.

L'Oréal Paris' commitment to bio-integrated skincare is evident in its recent marketing campaigns. For example, L'Oréal Paris' "Your Skin, Your Science" campaign highlights the brand's commitment to using science-backed ingredients and technologies in its products.

L'Oréal Paris' innovative bio-integrated skincare products and technologies are changing how we think about skincare. By working with the skin's natural biology, L'Oréal Paris is helping people to achieve their skincare goals more effectively and efficiently.

Benefits of L'Oréal Paris' Bio-Integrated Skincare

L'Oréal Paris' bio-integrated skincare products offer a number of benefits, including:

1. Improved skin health: Bio-integrated skincare products are designed to work with the skin's natural biology to improve its health. This can lead to a number of benefits, such as reduced inflammation, improved hydration, and increased collagen production, thereby making the skin look fresh and youthful.
2. Reduced appearance of wrinkles and fine lines: Bio-integrated skincare products can help to reduce the appearance of wrinkles and fine lines by boosting collagen production and exfoliating the skin.
3. Improved skin tone and texture: Bio-integrated skincare products can help to improve skin tone and texture by reducing the appearance of age spots and hyperpigmentation.
4. Increased skin hydration: Bio-integrated skincare products can help to increase skin hydration by containing ingredients such as hyaluronic acid and squalene.

Who Should Use L'Oréal Paris' Bio-Integrated Skincare?

L'Oréal Paris' bio-integrated skincare products are suitable for people of all ages and skin types. However, they are especially beneficial for people who are looking to improve their skin's health, redce the appearance of wrinkles and fine lines, or improve their skin tone and texture.

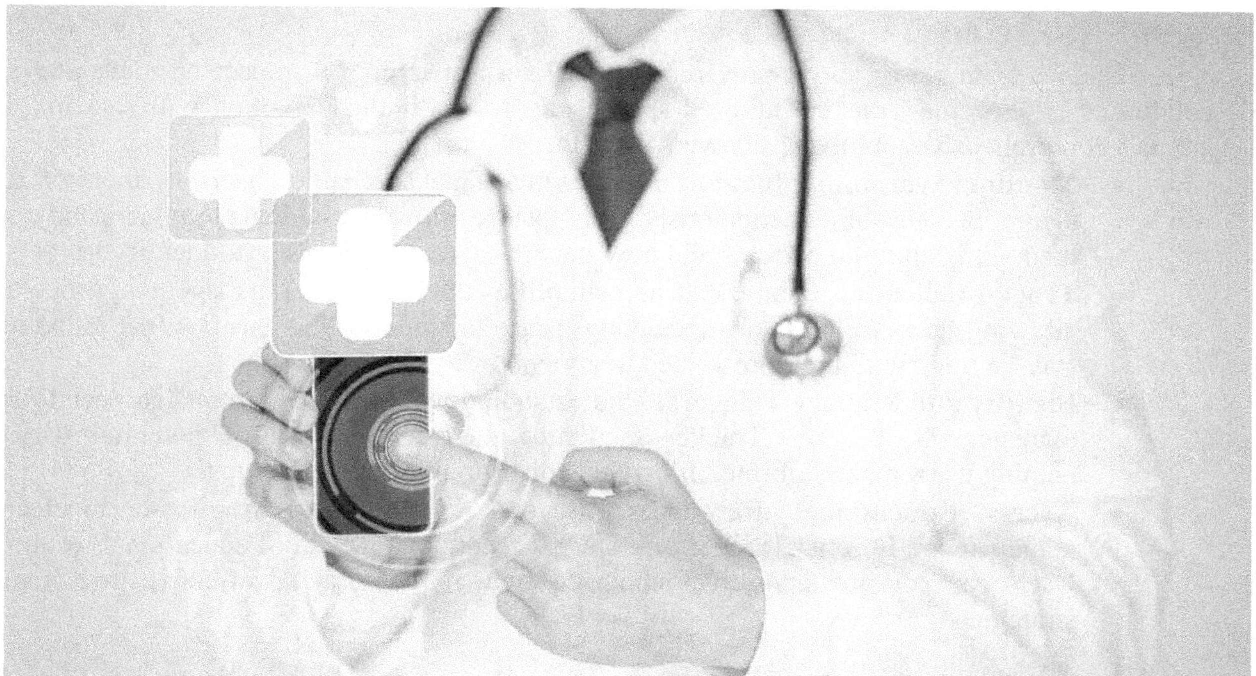

Chapter 7

AI Apps for Managing Skin Conditions

In an era characterized by technological advancements, AI-powered apps have emerged as indispensable allies in the realm of skincare, specifically for those managing various skin conditions. This chapter delves into the world of AI-powered apps, highlighting their pivotal role in assisting individuals dealing with skin conditions such as acne, eczema, and psoriasis.

The AI-Powered App Ecosystem for Skin Conditions:

In today's digital age, a plethora of AI-powered apps cater to the diverse needs of individuals facing skin conditions. These apps are designed to:

- **Inform Users About Their Skin Conditions:** AI-powered apps serve an abundance of knowledge, delivering comprehensive insights into specific skin conditions. Clients can access reliable information about their skin condition, enabling them to understand better its nature, triggers, and potential management strategies.

- **Personalize Treatment and Care:** Perhaps the most remarkable feature of these apps is their ability to offer personalized recommendations for treatment and care. Each user's experience is tailored to their unique skin profile, ensuring that the guidance aligns perfectly with their specific skin needs.

Real-Life Example: Eczema Tracker

A standout example of an AI-powered app making a meaningful impact on managing skin conditions is "Eczema Tracker" tailored specifically for individuals dealing with eczema, this app is a comprehensive tool that empowers users to:

- **Monitor Symptom Fluctuations:** Eczema Tracker enables users to monitor their symptoms over time meticulously. This feature allows individuals to understand better their skin condition patterns and how it evolves, making it easier to identify triggers.
- **Track Medication Usage:** The app simplifies the medication management process by allowing users to log their medication usage accurately. This ensures that individuals stay on track with their prescribed treatments.
- **Identify and Manage Triggers:** Understanding what worsens eczema is crucial for its management. Eczema Tracker facilitates the identification of potential triggers, helping users make informed lifestyle choices to minimize flare-ups.
- **Access Educational Resources:** Beyond symptom tracking and medication management, Eczema Tracker offers users access to a wealth of educational resources. Users can educate themselves about eczema, its causes, and effective management strategies.

The Value of AI-Powered Apps for Skin Conditions:

AI-powered apps bring plenty of benefits to individuals managing skin conditions:

- **Information Accessibility:** These apps democratize information, granting users easy access to valuable insights about their condition. Users can educate themselves and become informed advocates for their own skin health.
- **Supportive Community:** Many AI-powered apps foster a sense of community among users, allowing them to connect with others facing similar challenges. This sense of belonging can be invaluable for emotional support and shared experiences.
- **Personal Empowerment:** By tailoring recommendations and treatment plans to individual needs, AI-powered apps empower users to manage their skin conditions actively. This sense of control can significantly improve their quality of life.

In conclusion, AI-powered apps have revolutionized the management of skin conditions. These digital companions offer a treasure trove of knowledge, personalized guidance, and a sense of community for individuals navigating the complexities of skin health. As the AI app ecosystem continues to expand, the future holds even greater potential for enhanced support and empowerment for those dealing with skin conditions.

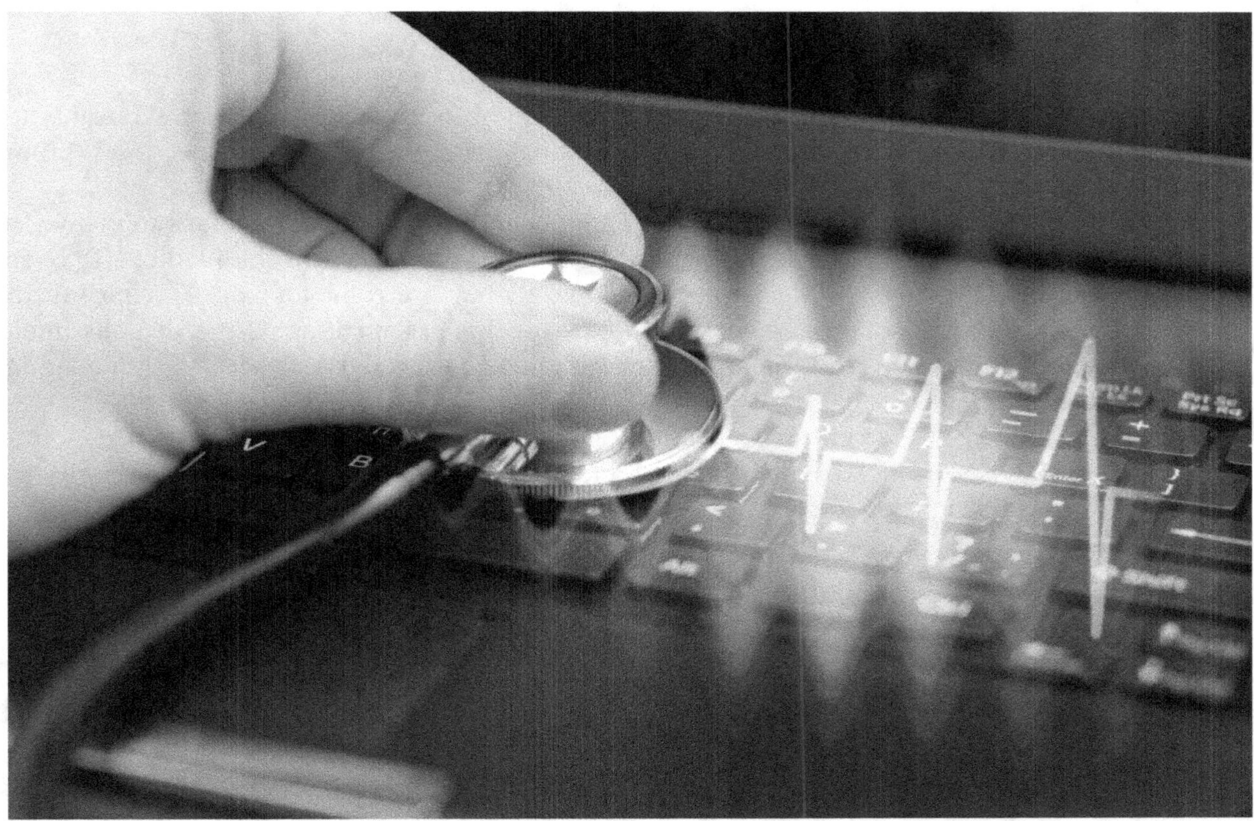

Chapter 8

Staying Ahead in the AI Beauty Landscape

Predictions and trends for the upcoming decade

The next decade promises unparalleled advancements in the AI beauty domain. We'll likely see AI tools becoming mainstream, with a focus on holistic health, where skincare, nutrition, and wellness intersect, all orchestrated by intelligent algorithms.

The role of quantum computing and advanced AI in beauty

Quantum computing, with its immense computational power, will take AI's capabilities in beauty to new heights. Tasks that take current computers years to compute might be accomplished in seconds, allowing for skincare solutions that adapt in real-time to changing environments and health conditions.

Tips for continuous learning and staying updated

In the fast-evolving landscape of AI beauty, continuous learning is crucial. Subscribing to relevant journals, attending tech-beauty conferences, and participating in online forums can help enthusiasts and professionals, such as dermatologists alike, stay abreast of the latest developments.

Advocating for responsible AI adoption in beauty

As with any technology, responsible adoption is key. It is crucial to approach AI beauty tools carefully, understand their capabilities and limitations, ensure ethical use, and promote transparency and fairness in AI-driven decisions.

You should be open to trying new devices and technologies. As AI continues to evolve, new and innovative skincare products and treatments will be introduced to the market. Be open to trying these new products and technologies to see if they are right for you. Having said that, consulting with a dermatologist or skincare professional is essential, as AI is still in its infancy. One cannot rely solely on it for diagnosis and treatments, especially for serious skin conditions like skin cancer.

In 2021, around 80 percent of Generation Z consumers in North America trusted Artificial Intelligence advisors for skincare products and routine recommendations. Gen Z was more trusting of AI advisors than the older generations..

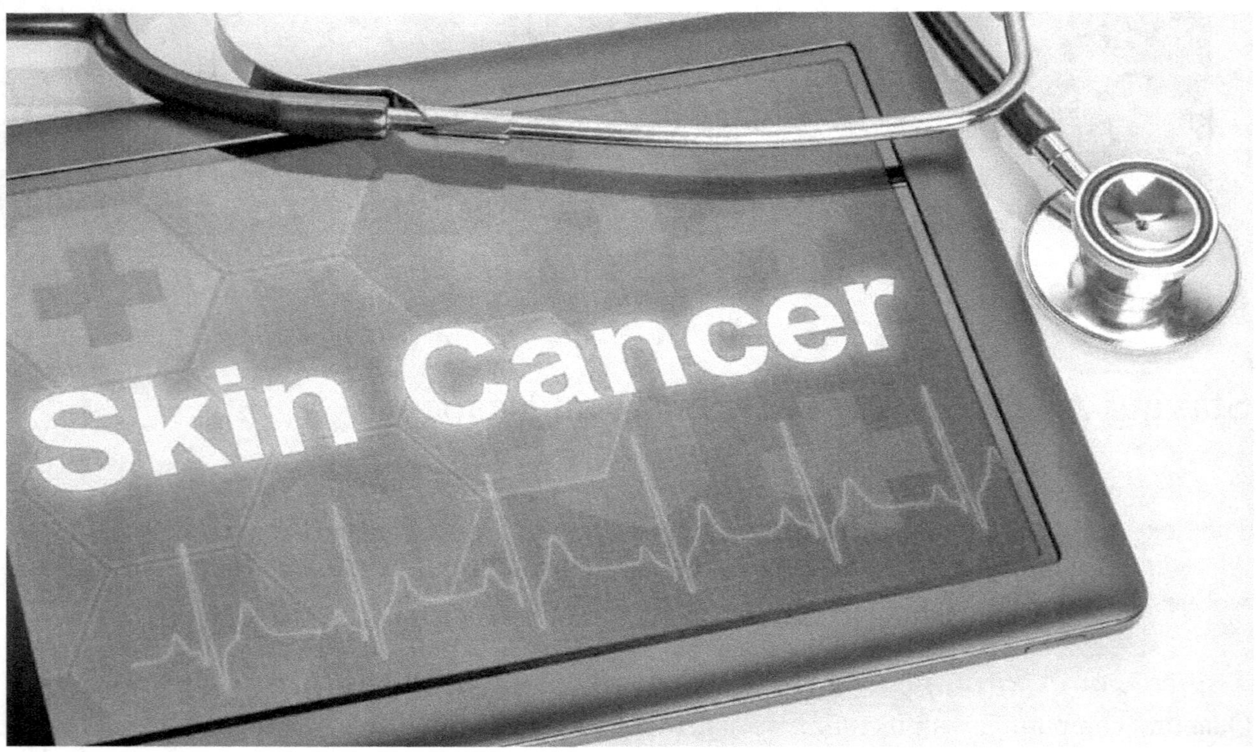

Chapter 9

AI-Based Diagnostic Tool for Skin Conditions

With approximately 2 billion people globally affected by at least one skin condition, these potential health and aesthetic concerns represent a significant source of morbidity. Notably, diagnostic accuracy for skin conditions improves significantly when conducted by dermatologists, leading to superior clinical outcomes compared to nonspecialist examinations. However, only 28% of skin-related cases are evaluated by specialists due to limited access to dermatological expertise. As a result, nonspecialist healthcare practitioners are vital in the initial assessment of skin lesions, initiating clinical management, and facilitating referrals. Still, research indicates that the diagnostic accuracy of nonspecialists ranges from 24% to 70%, emphasizing the need for resources like dermatology textbooks, medical portals, and online image search engines to offer more thorough guidance to nonspecialists.

To address this gap, various algorithms using Artificial Intelligence (AI) have been introduced, aiming to assist in interpreting both clinical and dermoscopic images of diverse skin conditions. A crucial question arises: can AI support primary care physicians (PCPs) and other specialists in diagnosing skin conditions from clinical images taken without specialized equipment?

This question was explored in a diagnostic study that incorporated multiple readers and cases. An innovative AI-driven tool was developed and assessed for clinical use. This study involved primary care physicians and nurse practitioners (NPs), who retrospectively examined cases spanning 120 distinct skin conditions. To ensure robust evaluation, a randomized approach ensured each professional reviewed every case both with and without AI assistance. The review occurred from February 21 to April 28, 2020, and data analysis ran from May 26, 2020, to January 27, 2021. The study's primary goal was to evaluate the efficacy of AI in improving diagnostic accuracy in dermatology.

In this study involving 20 primary care physicians and 20 nurse practitioners, a retrospective analysis of 1048 cases was conducted to determine AI's impact on diagnostic accuracy. The results showed a significant improvement in diagnostic agreement with a panel of dermatologists when AI was utilized. Therefore, involving experienced dermatologists in AI tool development can bolster primary care physicians and nonspecialists in accurately diagnosing dermatological cases with AI assistance.

Among PCPs, the use of AI increased diagnostic accuracy from 48% to 58%. Similarly, NPs saw an increase from 46% to 58% with AI integration. These results highlight AI's value in enhancing diagnostic accuracy, representing a significant stride in healthcare. Most importantly, these results mean that roughly one in every eight to ten cases receives a more accurate diagnosis due to AI's inclusion, showcasing AI's potential to enhance patient care and outcomes in dermatology.

Case Study #1: AI Doubles Diagnostic Accuracy of Skin Conditions Among Patients With Skin of Color

This case study discusses that AI can double the diagnostic accuracy of skin conditions among patients with skin of color. The study, which was published in the Journal of the American Academy of Dermatology, found that AI was able to correctly identify skin conditions in 83% of patients with skin of color, compared to 41% for dermatologists.

The study used an AI system called DeepDerm. DeepDerm is a machine learning system that was trained on a dataset of over 1 million images of skin lesions. DeepDerm is able to identify over 200 different skin conditions, including skin cancer and acne.

The study found that DeepDerm was particularly effective at diagnosing skin conditions in patients with darker skin tones. This is because darker skin tones can make it more difficult for dermatologists to identify skin conditions.

The use of AI to diagnose skin conditions has the potential to improve the early detection of skin cancer among patients with skin of color. Early detection of skin cancer is essential for successful treatment.

Case Study #2: AI May Soon Be Able to Detect Skin Cancer Better Than Dermatologists

This case study discusses how AI is being developed to detect skin cancer more accurately than dermatologists. AI systems are able to learn from large datasets of images of skin lesions, and they can then be used to identify lesions that are suspicious for skin cancer.

One example of an AI system that is being developed to detect skin cancer is DermExpert. DermExpert was developed by a team of researchers at the University of California, San Francisco. DermExpert is trained on a dataset of over 350,000 images of skin lesions, and it can identify over 200 different skin conditions, including skin cancer.

In a study published in the Journal of the American Academy of Dermatology, DermExpert was shown to be more accurate than dermatologists at diagnosing melanoma, the most deadly type of skin cancer. The study found that DermExpert correctly identified 95% of melanomas, while dermatologists correctly identified only 87% of melanomas.

Another AI system that is being developed to detect skin cancer is Melanoma AI. Melanoma AI was developed by a team of researchers at Stanford University. Melanoma AI is trained on a dataset of over 1 million images of skin lesions, and it can identify melanoma with high accuracy.

In a study published in the journal Nature Medicine, Melanoma AI was shown to be more accurate than dermatologists at diagnosing melanoma. The study found that Melanoma AI correctly identified 99% of melanomas, while dermatologists correctly identified only 87% of melanomas.

The use of AI to detect skin cancer has the potential to improve the early detection of skin cancer. Early detection of skin cancer is essential for successful treatment.

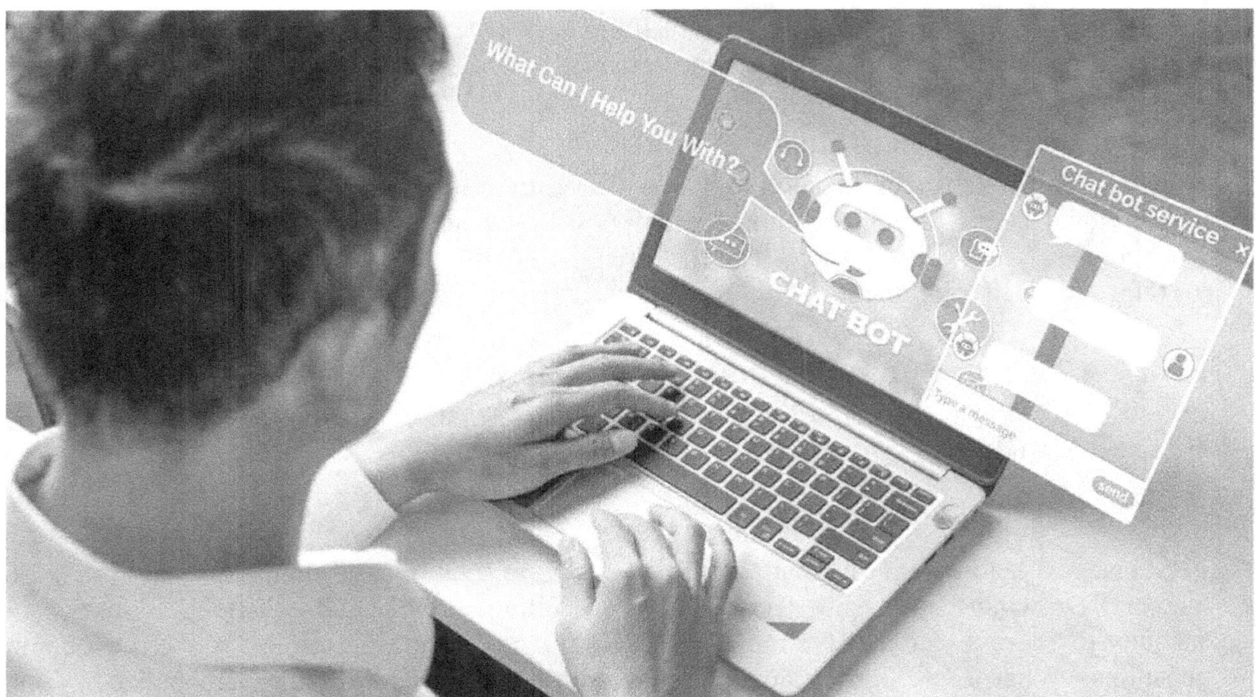

Chapter 10

AI Chatbots: Your On-Demand Skin Care Advisors

In today's fast-paced world, where convenience and accessibility are paramount, AI chatbots have emerged as invaluable tools in the realm of skincare. This chapter explores in greater detail how AI chatbots are revolutionizing the skincare industry by providing patients with on-demand, personalized skin care advice.

The Multifaceted Role of AI Chatbots in Skincare:

AI chatbots are a game-changer in the world of skincare, offering a multifaceted approach to patient care and education. They serve as versatile tools capable of:

Answering Patient Questions with Precision:

AI chatbots are equipped to respond to a vast array of patient inquiries, spanning questions related to skin conditions, treatment options, and product recommendations. Patients can now receive accurate and relevant information at their fingertips, eliminating the need to sift through mountains of online resources or wait for a healthcare appointment.

Enlightening Patients About Skin Conditions:

Understanding one's skin condition is the first step toward effective treatment and self-care. AI chatbots play a pivotal role in providing patients with comprehensive knowledge about various skin conditions, including but not limited to acne, eczema, and psoriasis. With readily available information, people can become better informed about their own skin health.

Personalized Product Recommendations:

AI chatbots take personalization to the next level by recommending skincare products tailored to individual needs. These recommendations are based on analyzing the patient's unique skin type, concerns, and goals. Patients can trust that the products suggested are suitable and effective for their specific requirements.

Real-World Examples: AI Chatbots in Action

Let's delve into real-world examples of AI chatbots that are making a substantial impact on the skincare landscape:

Skinsei: Your Personalized Skincare Guru

Skinsei, a leading AI chatbot, stands as a prime example of innovation in the skincare industry. Drawing from a vast dataset of over 1 million skin-related questions, Skinsei has the capacity to address an extensive range of patient queries, from the simplest to the most complex questions. What sets Skinsei apart is its ability to provide highly personalized skincare recommendations, creating a truly tailored experience for each user.

American Academy of Dermatology (AAD): Guiding Your Skin Health

The AAD has developed an AI chatbot designed to empower patients with knowledge about skin conditions. This chatbot fields questions on conditions like acne, eczema, and psoriasis, offering reliable and evidence-based information. Patients can access insights on skincare treatments and products, all from a reputable source within the dermatology field.

The Advantages of AI Chatbots in Skincare:

AI chatbots are transforming the skincare landscape by offering distinct benefits to patients:
24/7 Availability: One of the standout benefits of AI chatbots is their round-the-clock availability. Patients can get help whenever they need it, regardless of the time or day, ensuring that skin concerns are addressed promptly.

Confidentiality and Comfort:

AI chatbots provide a confidential and non-judgmental space for patients to discuss their skincare questions and concerns. This privacy encourages open dialogue, helping patients feel more at ease when seeking guidance on personal skin issues.

A More Accessible Skincare Future:

In conclusion, AI chatbots can democratize skincare by making it accessible to everyone at any convenient time. These digital assistants offer convenient, reliable, and personalized information and advice. Patients are empowered to take charge of their skincare journey, armed with the knowledge and recommendations needed to achieve healthy and radiant skin. As the integration of AI in skincare continues to evolve, the future holds even more tremendous promise for accessible and efficient skincare solutions.

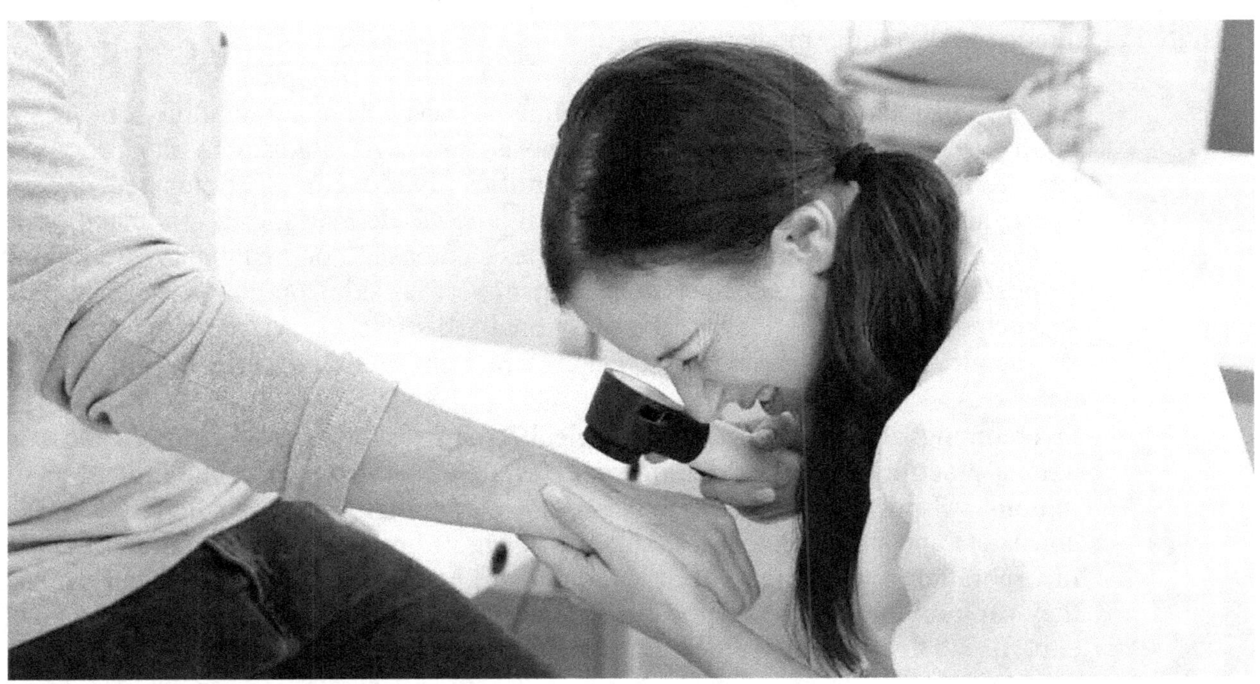

Chapter 11

AI and Dermatoscopy

Dermatoscopy, also known as Dermoscopy or epiluminescence microscopy, is a non-invasive imaging technique that allows dermatologists to examine skin lesions in detail. When coupled with AI, dermatoscopy becomes an even more powerful tool for identifying skin types, detecting skin disorders, improving patient outcomes, and advancing the field of dermatology and skincare.

Enhanced Accuracy in Skin Type Analysis and Skin Lesion Diagnosis

Dermatoscopy, by itself, is a valuable technique that allows dermatologists to visualize skin lesions at a magnified level. However, the interpretation of dermatoscopic images can be challenging, relying on the dermatologist's expertise and experience. AI algorithms, particularly deep learning models, have shown remarkable promise in analyzing these images with exceptional accuracy.

When fed with large datasets of dermatoscopic images, AI systems can learn to recognize patterns and structures indicative of various skin types and conditions, including melanoma, basal cell carcinoma, and squamous cell carcinoma. These algorithms can highlight suspicious features, helping dermatologists make more accurate and timely diagnoses and identify skin types or diseases. A dermatoscope, when coupled with AI, can also identify skin types by meticulously examining the skin structure and subsequently advise the best possible products suited to an individual's requirements.

- Faster Diagnosis and Reduced Waiting Times: The integration of AI with dermatoscopy also leads to faster diagnosis times. AI algorithms can process and analyze dermatoscopic images rapidly, significantly reducing the time needed to reach a diagnosis. This speed is crucial, as it allows dermatologists to make prompt decisions regarding the need for further tests, biopsies, or treatments. Additionally, reduced waiting times can alleviate patient anxiety, as skin conditions, especially those suspected to be cancerous, can be emotionally distressing. AI can help expedite the diagnostic process, leading to quicker treatment initiation and improved patient outcomes.
- Overcoming Variability in Dermatological Expertise: Dermatology expertise can vary among practitioners, and access to specialized dermatologists may be limited in some regions. AI-powered dermatoscopy provides a solution to this challenge by offering consistent and standardized assessments. AI algorithms are trained on diverse datasets, incorporating a wide range of dermatological knowledge and experience. As a result, they can provide reliable diagnostic support irrespective of the dermatologist's level of expertise. This democratization of dermatological expertise is particularly valuable in remote or underserved areas where access to dermatological specialists may be limited. AI-assisted dermatoscopy can serve as a valuable tool for general practitioners and healthcare providers, enabling them to make more informed decisions about patient referrals and treatment plans.

In conclusion, the union of AI and dermatoscopy represents a significant leap forward in the field of dermatology. By enhancing the analysis of skin type identification, accuracy of skin lesion diagnosis, reducing waiting times, standardizing expertise, improving screening and follow-up care, and facilitating research, AI-powered dermatoscopy is poised to revolutionize the way skin conditions are diagnosed and managed. It empowers dermatologists with valuable insights, ultimately leading to better patient outcomes and a brighter future for dermatological healthcare.

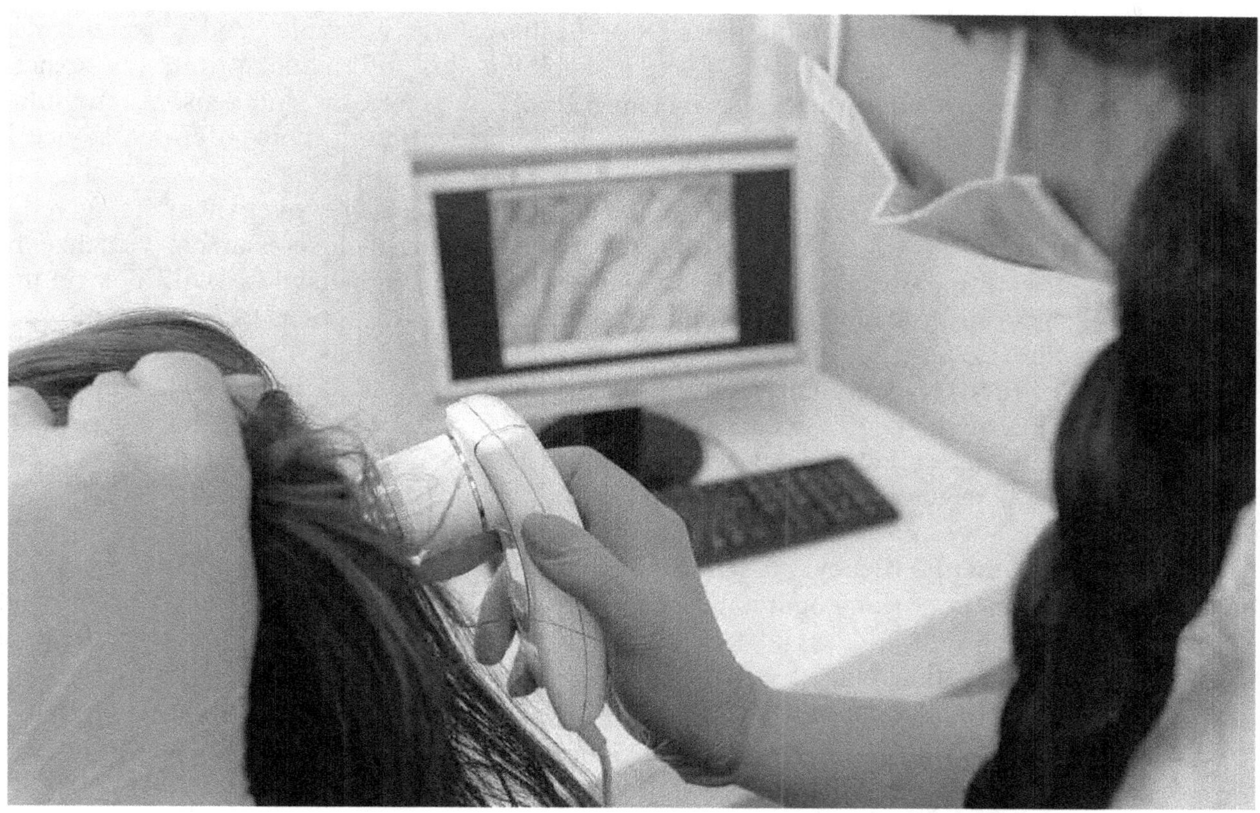

Chapter 12

Top 10 Advantages of AI in Dermatology and Beauty

1. **Early Detection of Skin Conditions:** AI systems are trained at pattern recognition. By training on vast databases of skin condition images, these systems can identify even subtle changes or anomalies that might be indicative of skin diseases or cancers. Early detection can lead to early intervention, which is particularly crucial for conditions like melanoma, where timely treatment can be lifesaving.
2. **Consistency in Diagnosis:** Every dermatologist brings their own unique experiences and biases to a diagnosis. While this expertise is invaluable, it can sometimes lead to inconsistencies. AI can provide a consistent analysis grounded in the vast amount of data it has been trained on by experienced skin specialists, offering a reliable benchmark that professionals can use as a reference.
3. **Personalized Skincare Recommendations:** Everyone's skin is unique, requiring different care regimens and products. AI can assess factors such as skin type, tone, and problem areas to provide tailored skincare advice. This individualized approach can lead to better results, as it targets each person's specific needs and challenges.
4. **Cost-Effectiveness:** Initial screenings or consultations can be time-consuming and expensive. AI-driven preliminary screenings can help streamline the process, reducing the cost for patients and clinics alike. This not only makes dermatological care more affordable but also allows professionals to prioritize and focus on more complex cases.

5. **Data Integration:** With the rise of health-centric wearables and apps, there is a plethora of data available. AI can combine this information, from UV exposure tracked by smartwatches to moisture levels measured by skin sensors, providing a holistic view of an individual's skin health and offering more informed advice and treatment options.

6. **Virtual Try-Ons:** Shopping for beauty products can be overwhelming, given the sheer variety available. AI-powered virtual try-ons help consumers visualize how different products—such as lipsticks, eyeshadows, or hairstyles—will look on them. This leads to more confident purchasing decisions and reduces the chances of product returns.

7. **Product Development:** Consumer needs and preferences are ever-evolving. AI can sift through reviews, feedback, and market trends to pinpoint consumers' desires. This intelligence allows beauty companies to innovate and release products that are more in tune with current market demands.

8. **Treatment Efficacy:** AI can serve as an invaluable tool in tracking the progression or regression of skin conditions. Consistently analyzing skin over time can offer insights into the effectiveness of treatments, enabling dermatologists to adjust strategies for optimal patient outcomes.

9. **Continual Learning:** The field of dermatology is dynamic, with new research and findings emerging regularly. AI models can continually update and refine their knowledge, ensuring that their advice and analyses are based on the latest and most accurate information.

10. **Accessibility:** Not everyone can access dermatological care easily, especially in remote or underserved regions. AI-driven apps and platforms can bridge this gap, offering individuals preliminary assessments, advice, and the means to connect with professionals when needed.

Incorporating AI into the realms of dermatology and beauty offers a blend of efficiency, personalization, and accessibility, indicating a new era of care and consumer experience. However, the symbiotic relationship between AI and human expertise remains paramount for success. Hence, we always need an experienced dermatologist and a team of AI experts to develop and update the AI tools and software so that the advice offered to the person is specifically tailored to meet the requirements of the concerned person.

Conclusion:

Summarizing the transformative potential of AI in skincare:

As we reach the conclusion, it is evident that AI's integration into skincare is not a fleeting trend but a transformative shift. It promises a future where skincare is not just personalized but predictive, where products and routines evolve in real time, and where beauty and health converge seamlessly.

Practical steps to embrace AI-powered skincare:

Embracing AI in skin care is not about discarding old routines but enhancing them. It is about leveraging technology for informed choices, using AI-driven insights to complement, not replace, expert advice, and approaching skincare with a balance of technology and touch.

Further resources and avenues to explore AI-Powered Skin Care:

For those eager to dive deeper, numerous resources, from online courses to dedicated forums, can help explore the fascinating world of AI-powered skincare. As we stand at the cusp of this revolution, the journey ahead promises to be one of discovery, innovation, and beauty in the truest sense.

References

US Virtual and Augmented Reality Users 2021, XR Use Expands Beyond Fun and Games, Report by Victoria Petrock | Apr 15, 2021

https://www.insiderintelligence.com/content/us-virtual-augmented-reality-users-2021

Loreal **Virtual Makeup try-on technology**

https://www.loreal.com/en/articles/science-and-technology/makeup-virtual-try-on-maybelline/

Sephora Virtual Artist
https://www.sephora.my/pages/virtual-artist

US beauty shoppers turn to websites, not department stores, when researching products

Article by Alexandra Samet | Sep 1, 2023

https://www.insiderintelligence.com/content/us-beauty-shoppers-turn-websites-not-department-stores-researching-products

Percentage of Gen Z consumers who trust AI advisors for personalized skincare recommendations in North America in 2021

https://www.statista.com/statistics/1289772/gen-z-s-trust-in-ai-beauty-advisors-in-north-america/